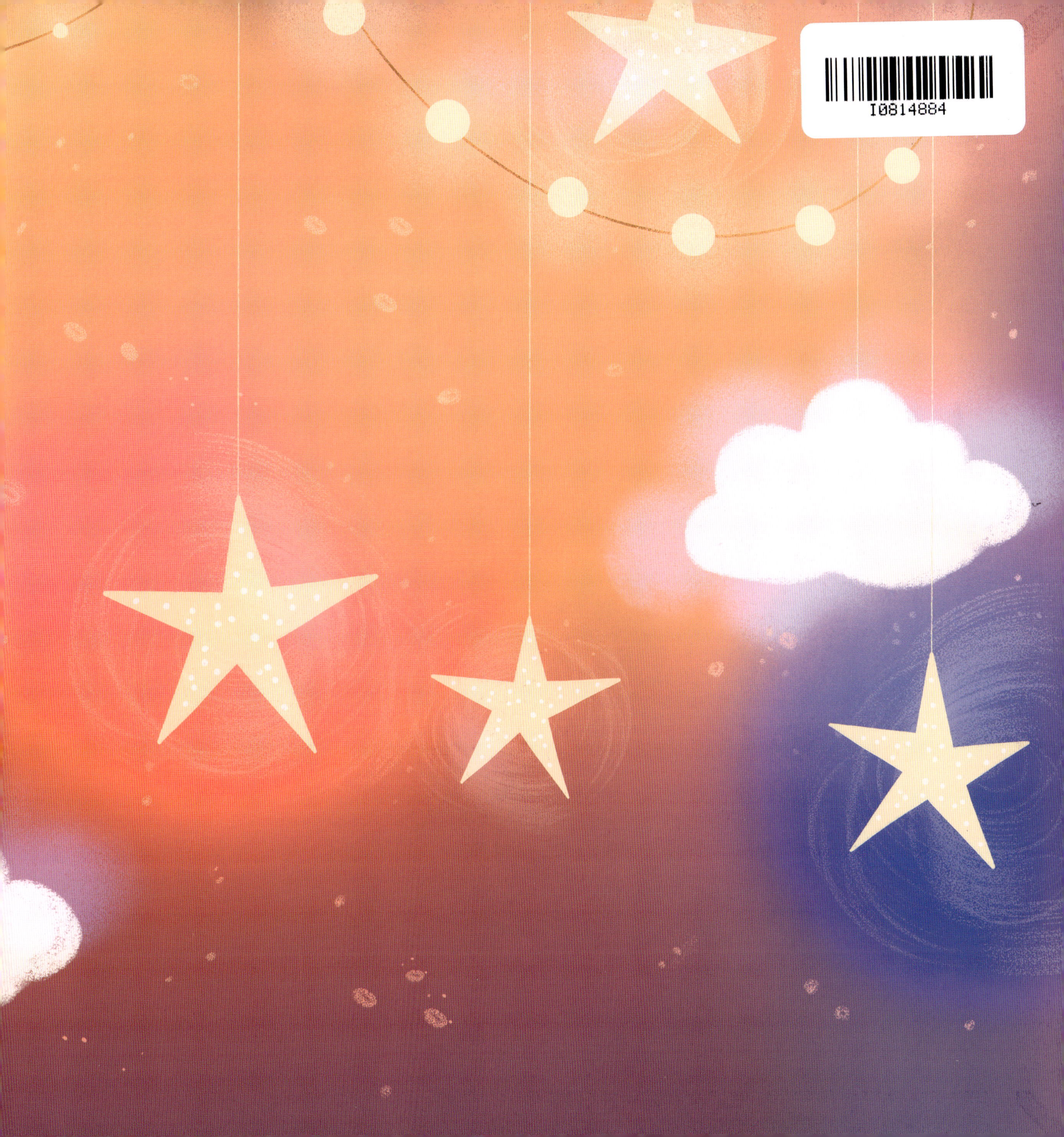

First published in Great Britain in 2024 by Starshine Books

SPCK Group
Studio 101
The Record Hall
16–16A Baldwin's Gardens
London EC1N 7RJ

www.spck.org.uk

Inspired by her own story of overcoming adversity, Katie Piper's The UnSeen is a publishing collection that sheds light on the untold stories of hope that deserve to be heard.

British Library Cataloguing-in-Publication Data

A catalogue record for this book is available from the British Library

ISBN 978-1-915749-23-9

1 2 3 4 5 6 7 8 9 10

Printed in China by Dream Colour (Hong Kong) Printing Ltd

Produced on paper from sustainable forests

STARSHINE BOOKS

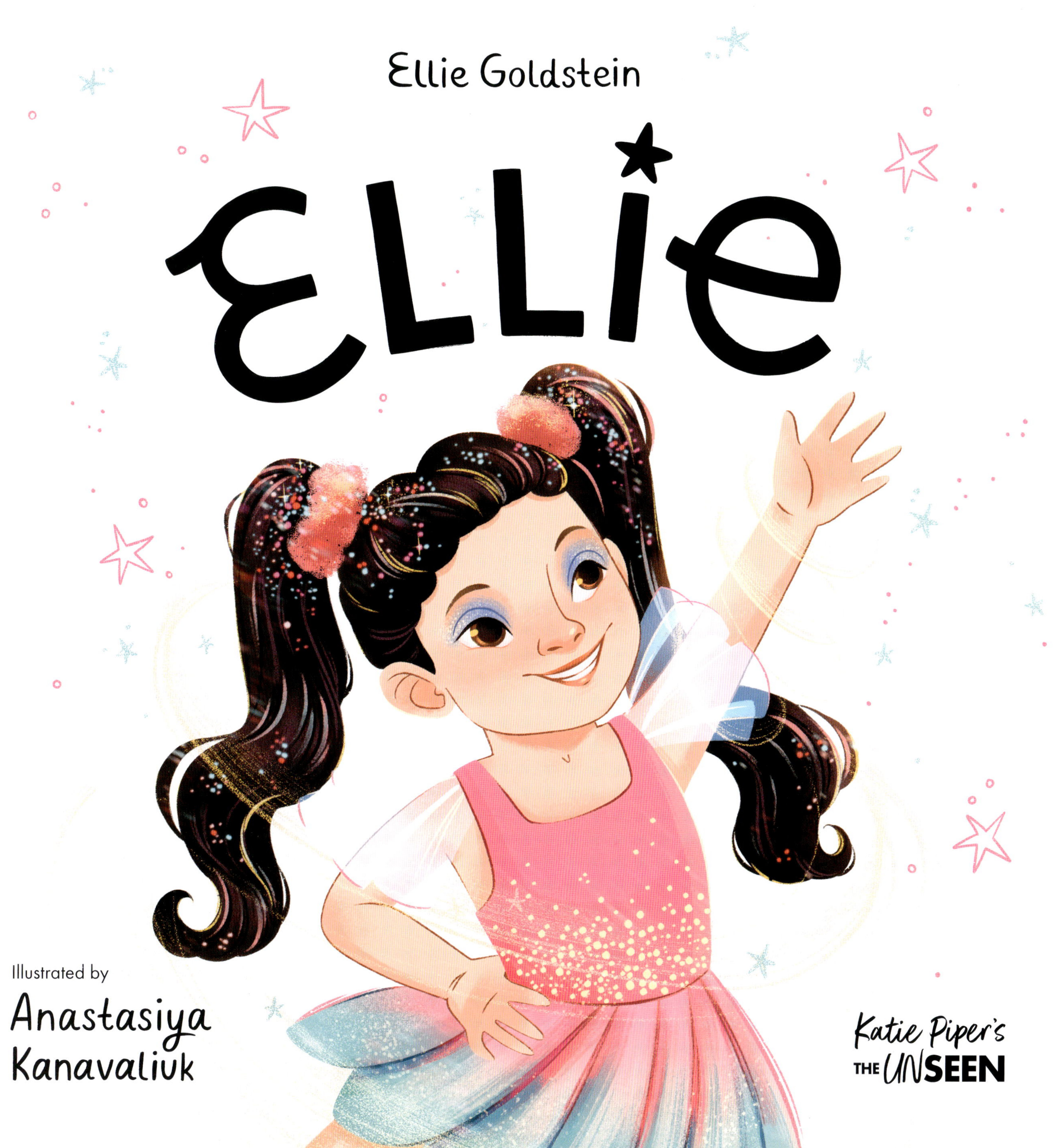
Ellie Goldstein
Ellie
Illustrated by
Anastasiya Kanavaliuk
Katie Piper's
THE UNSEEN

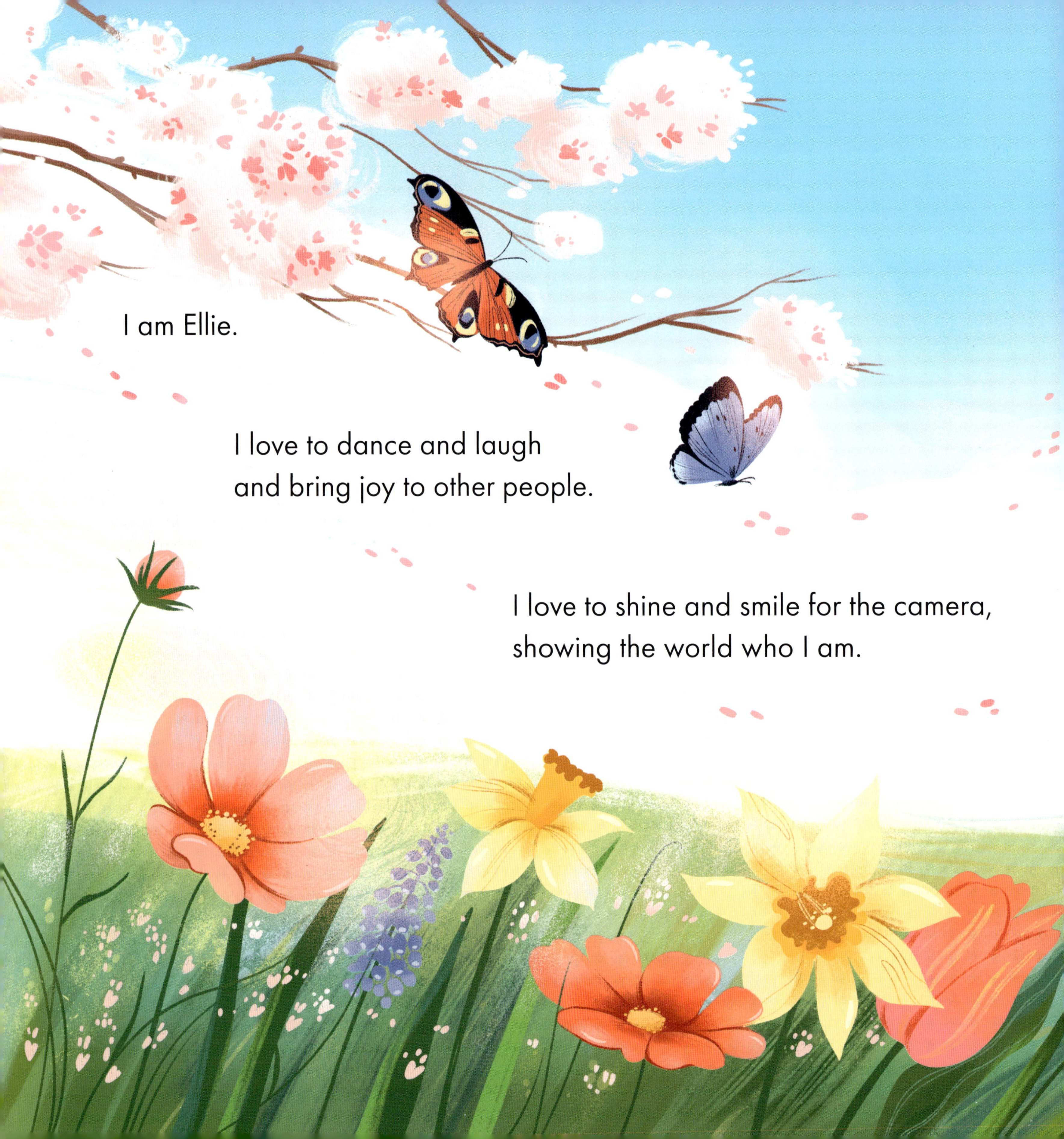

I am Ellie.

I love to dance and laugh
and bring joy to other people.

I love to shine and smile for the camera,
showing the world who I am.

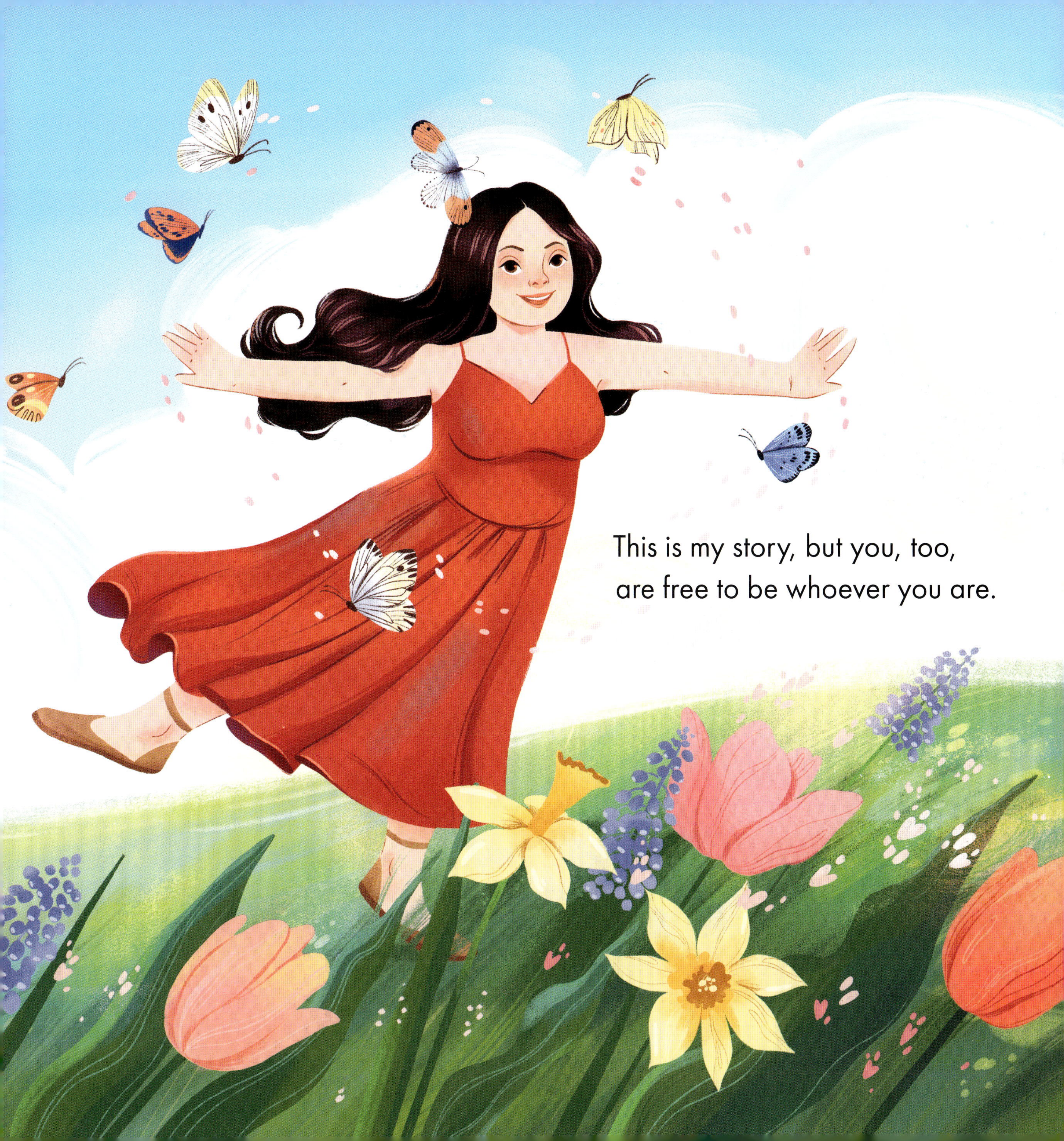

This is my story, but you, too,
are free to be whoever you are.

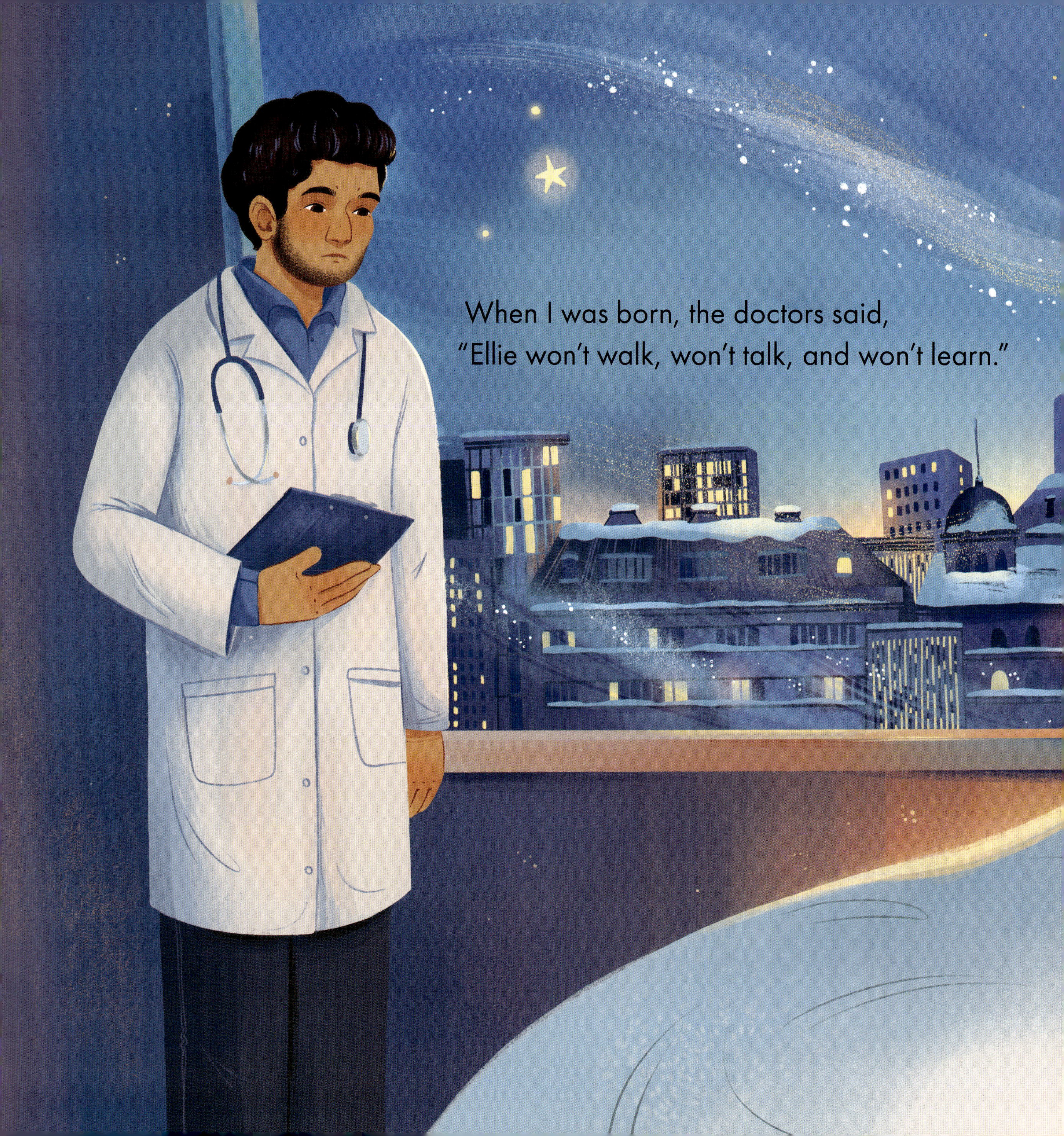

When I was born, the doctors said,
"Ellie won't walk, won't talk, and won't learn."

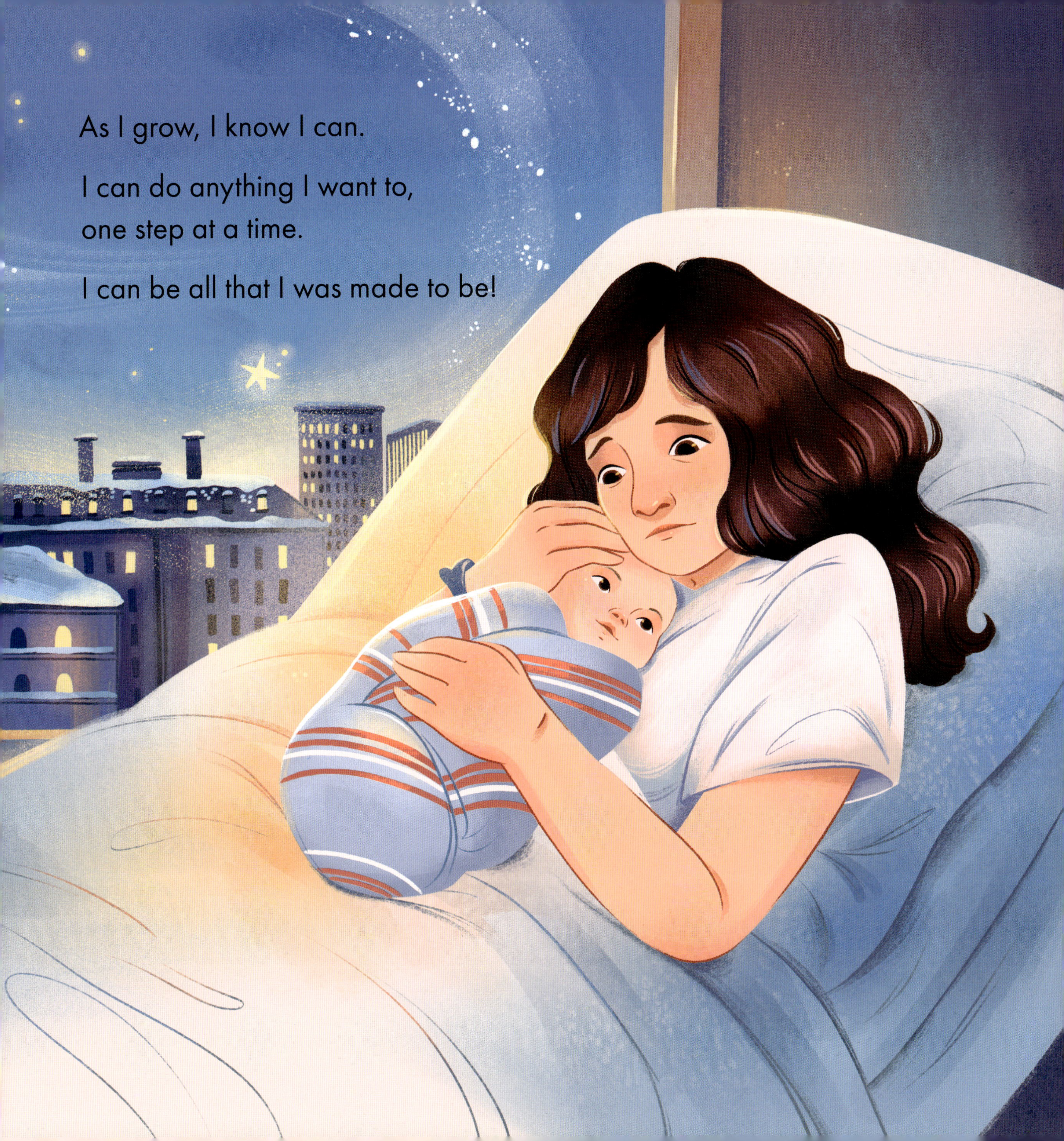

As I grow, I know I can.

I can do anything I want to,
one step at a time.

I can be all that I was made to be!

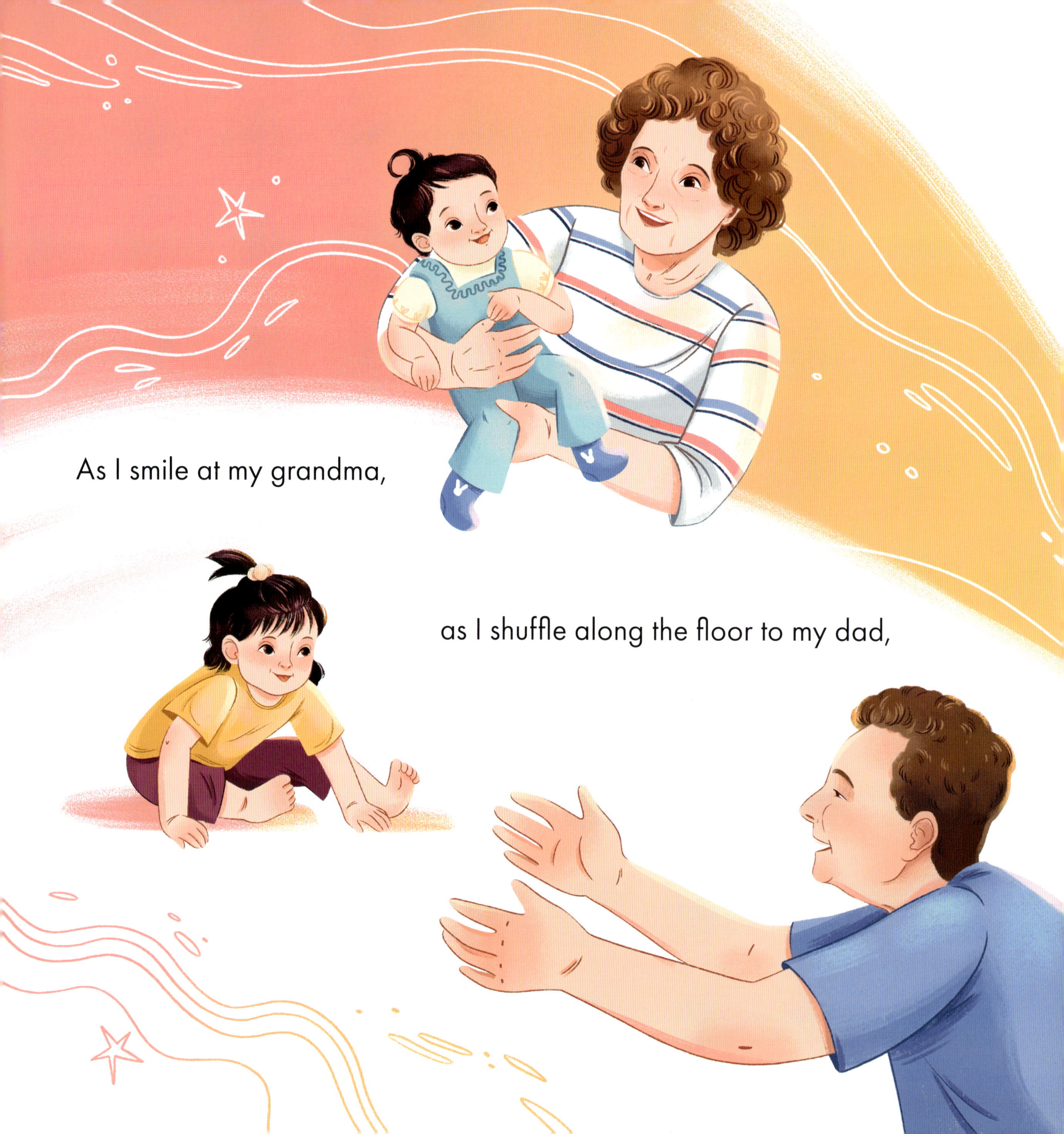

As I smile at my grandma,

as I shuffle along the floor to my dad,

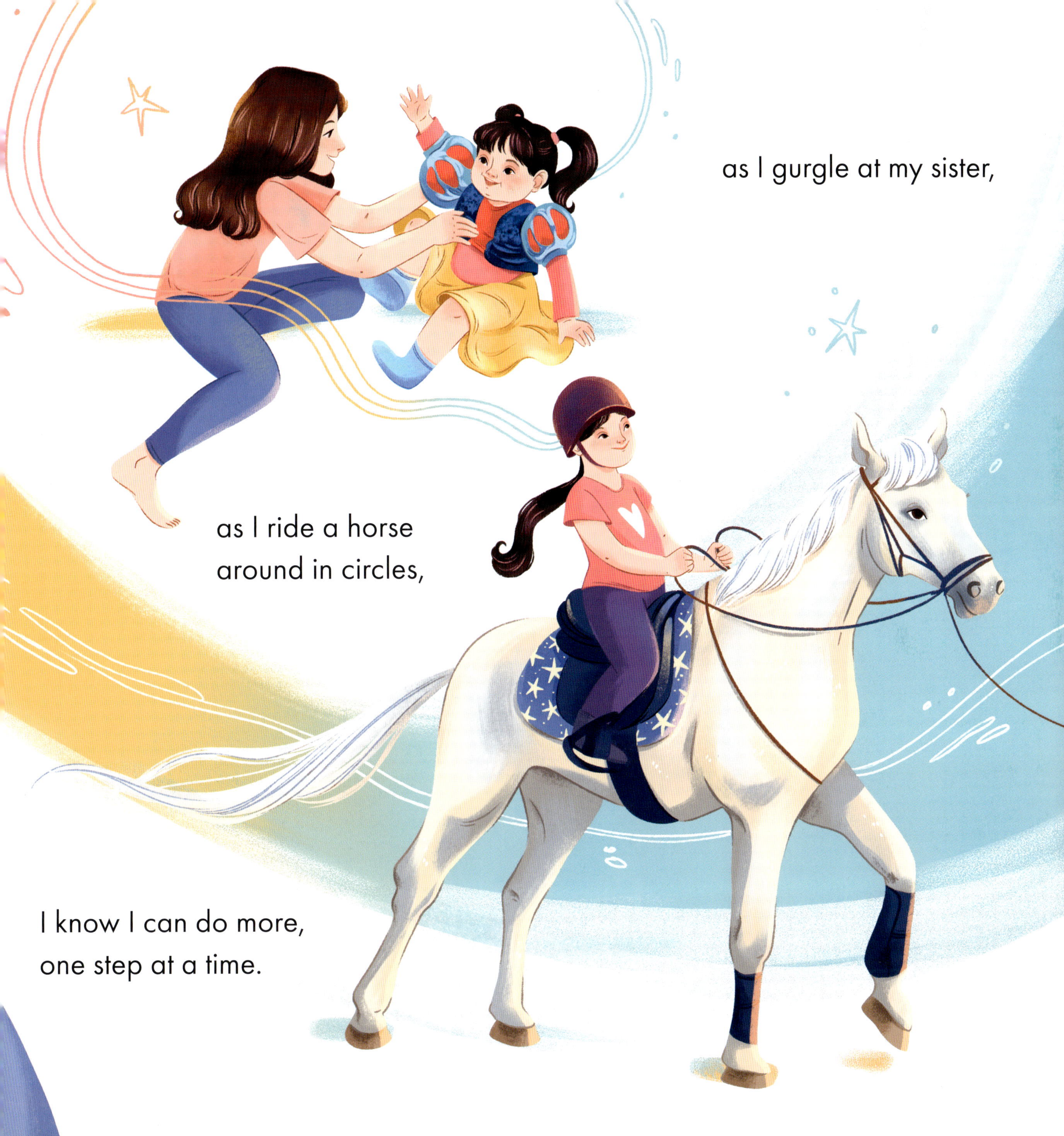

as I gurgle at my sister,

as I ride a horse
around in circles,

I know I can do more,
one step at a time.

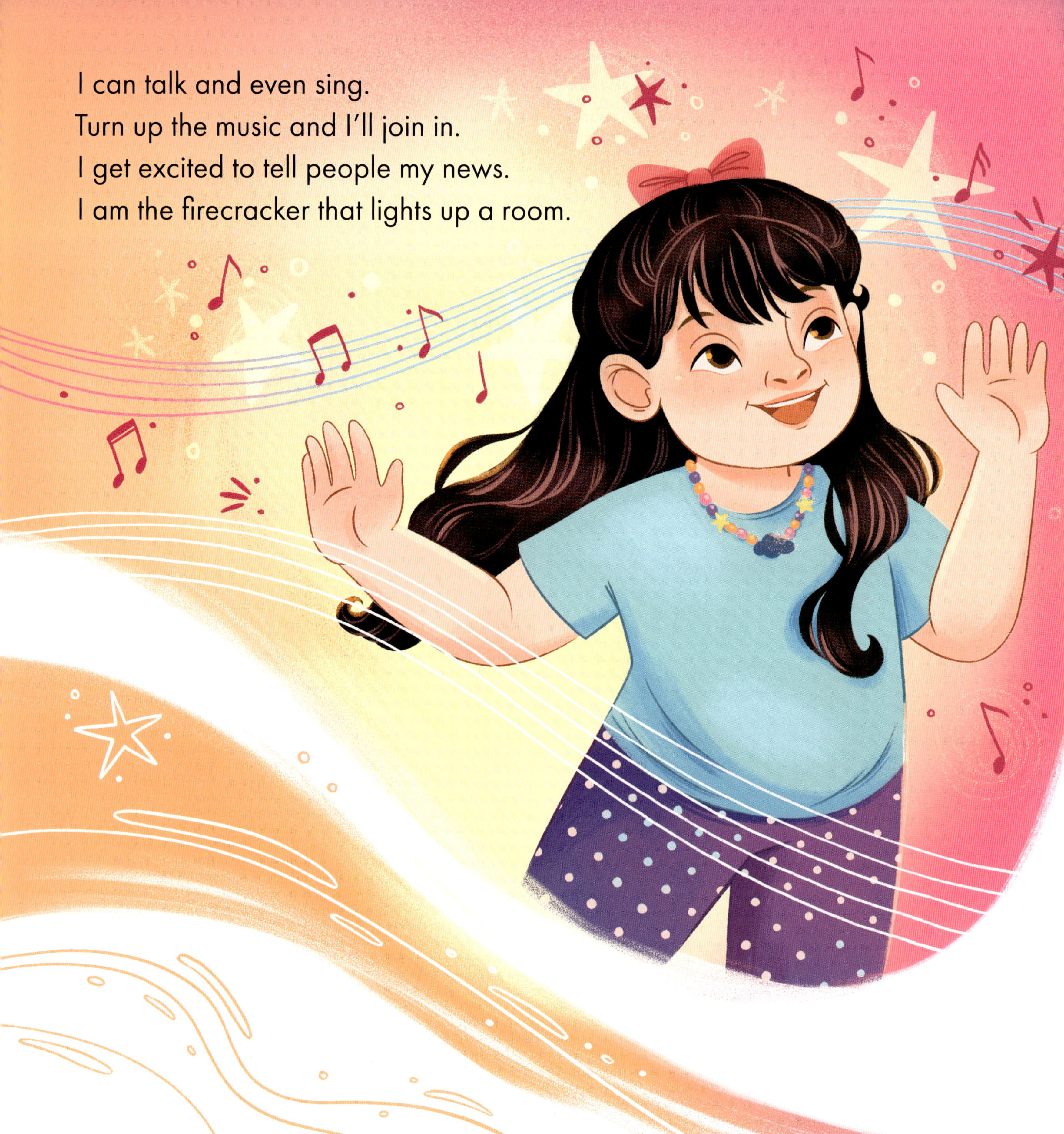

I can talk and even sing.
Turn up the music and I'll join in.
I get excited to tell people my news.
I am the firecracker that lights up a room.

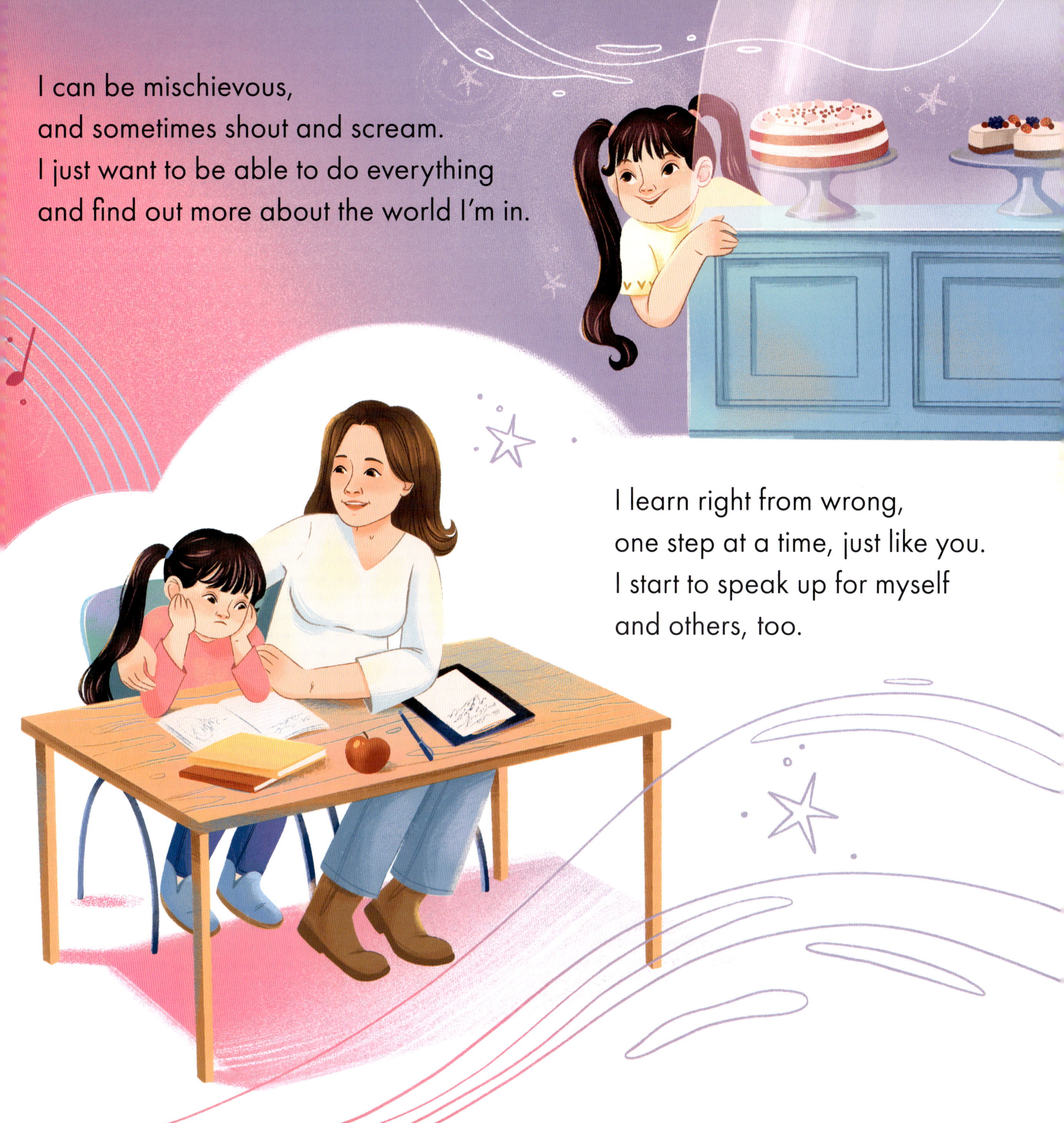

I can be mischievous,
and sometimes shout and scream.
I just want to be able to do everything
and find out more about the world I'm in.

I learn right from wrong,
one step at a time, just like you.
I start to speak up for myself
and others, too.

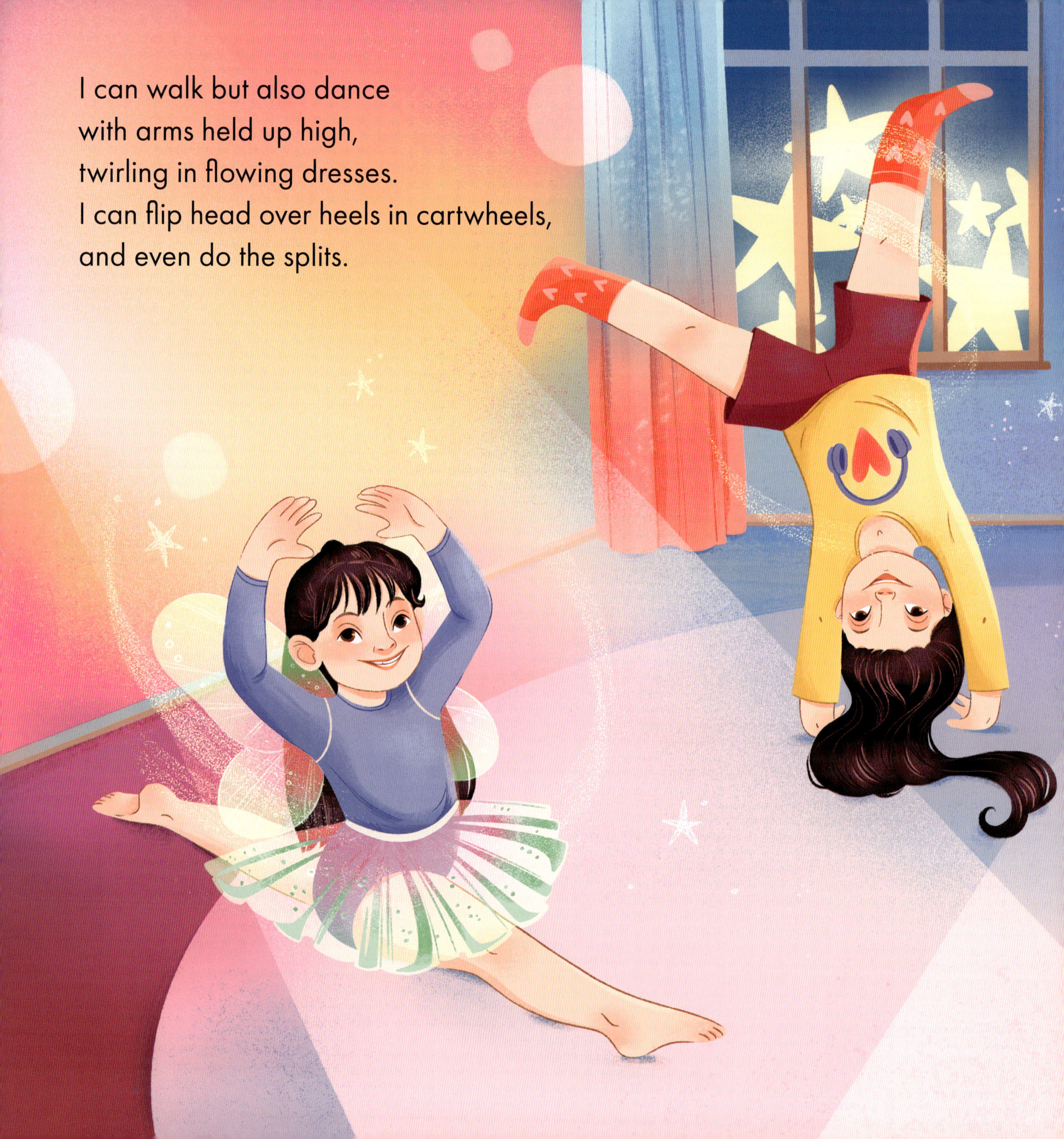

I can walk but also dance
with arms held up high,
twirling in flowing dresses.
I can flip head over heels in cartwheels,
and even do the splits.

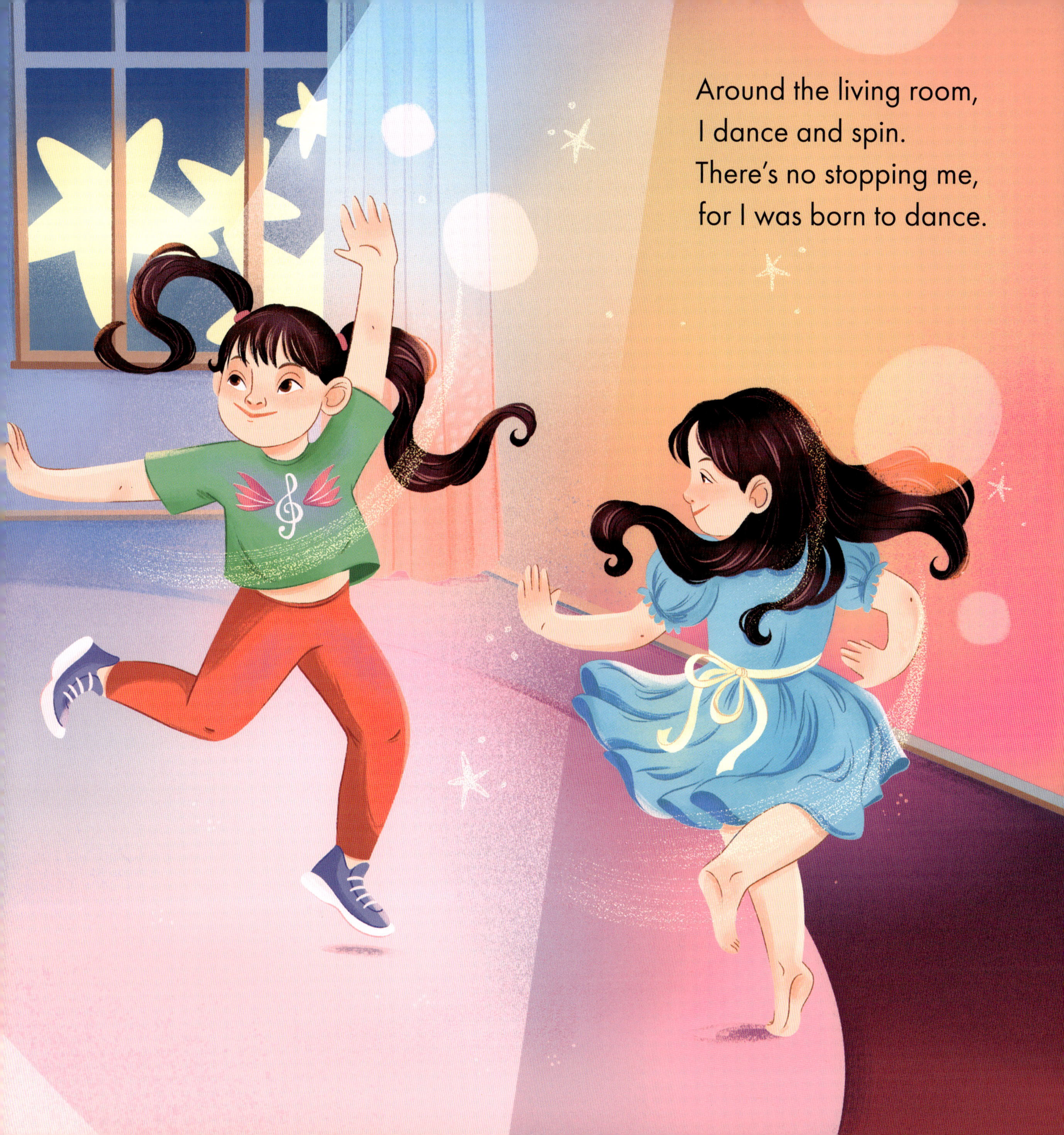

Around the living room,
I dance and spin.
There's no stopping me,
for I was born to dance.

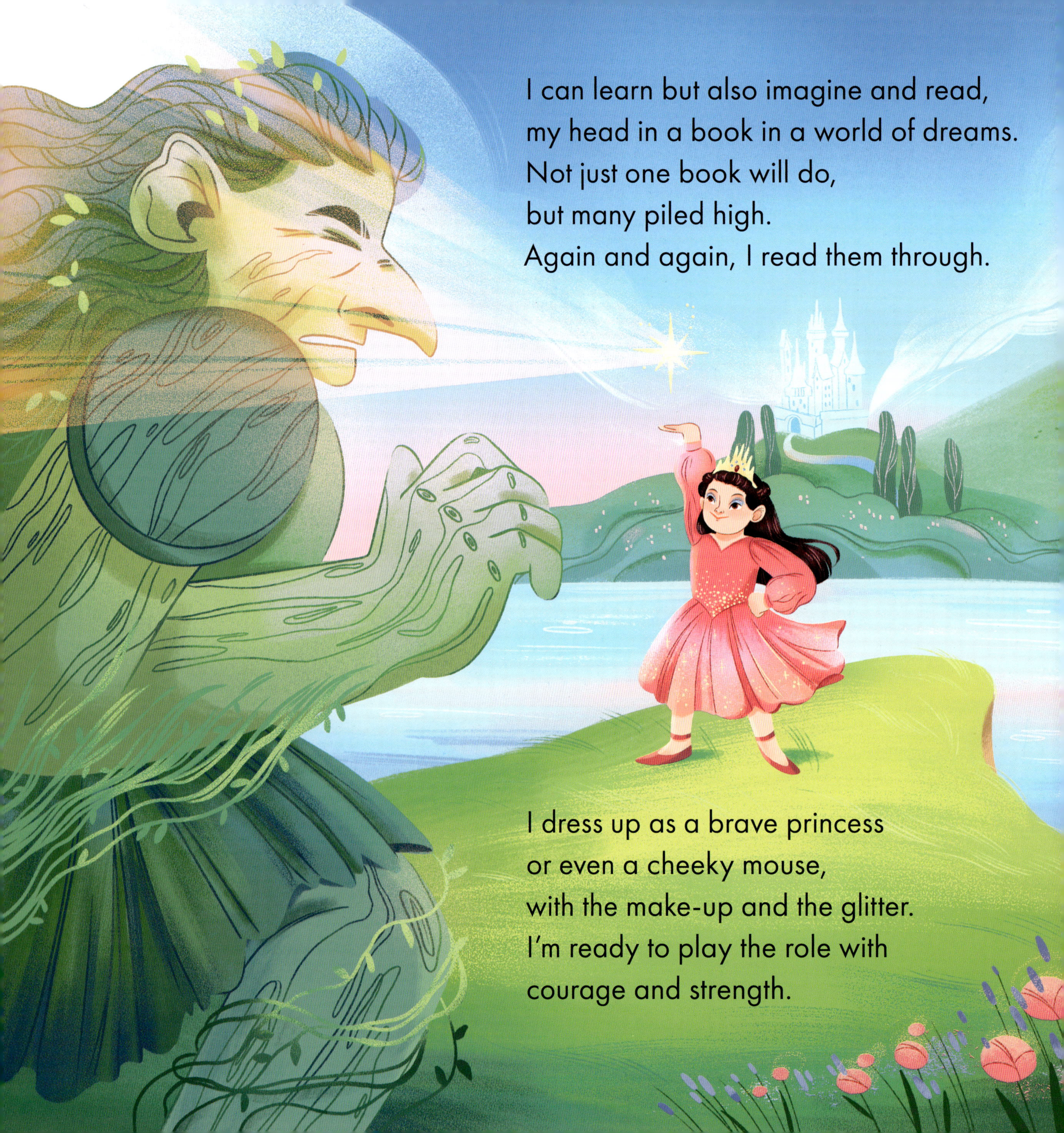

I can learn but also imagine and read,
my head in a book in a world of dreams.
Not just one book will do,
but many piled high.
Again and again, I read them through.

I dress up as a brave princess
or even a cheeky mouse,
with the make-up and the glitter.
I'm ready to play the role with
courage and strength.

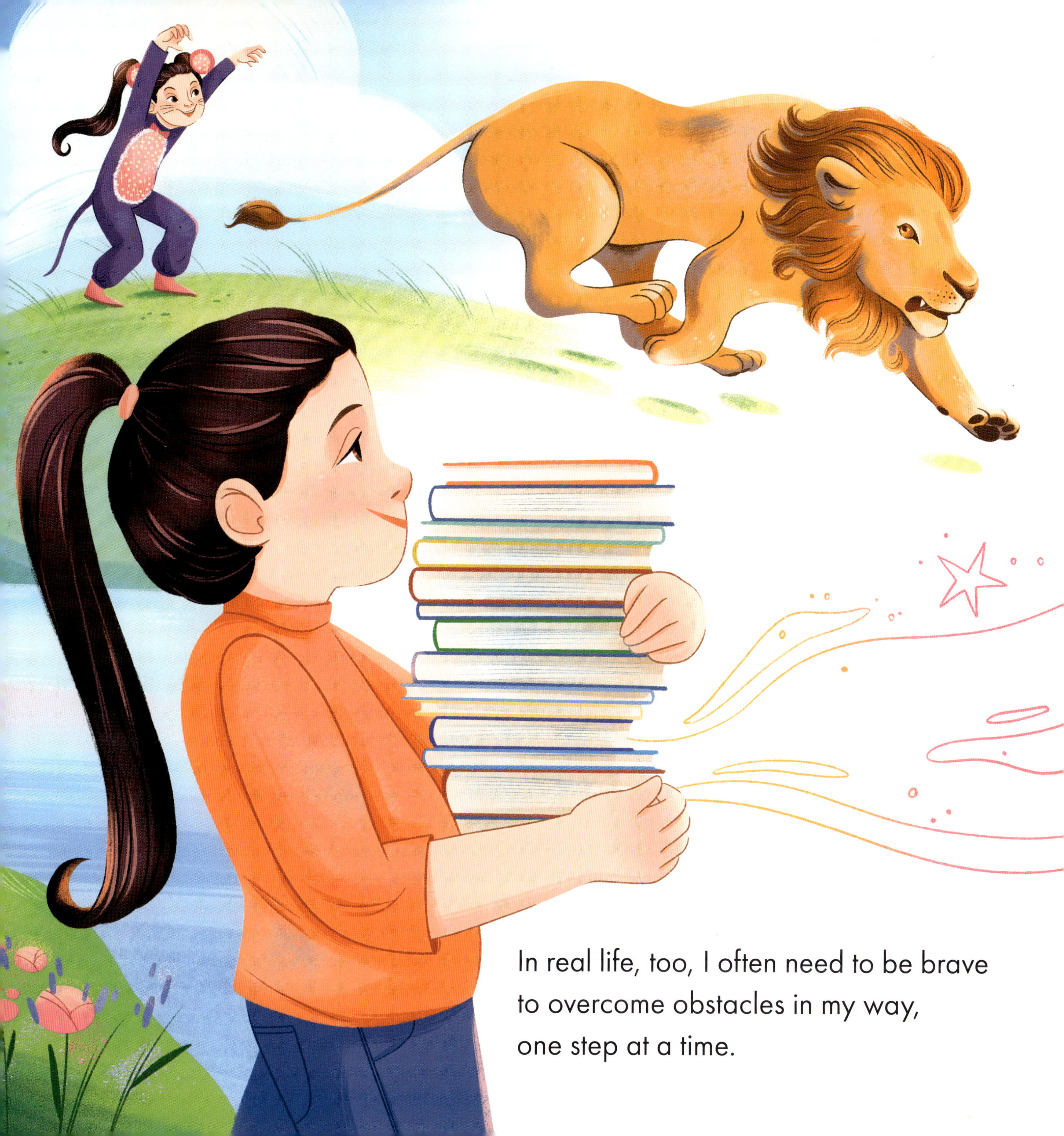

In real life, too, I often need to be brave to overcome obstacles in my way, one step at a time.

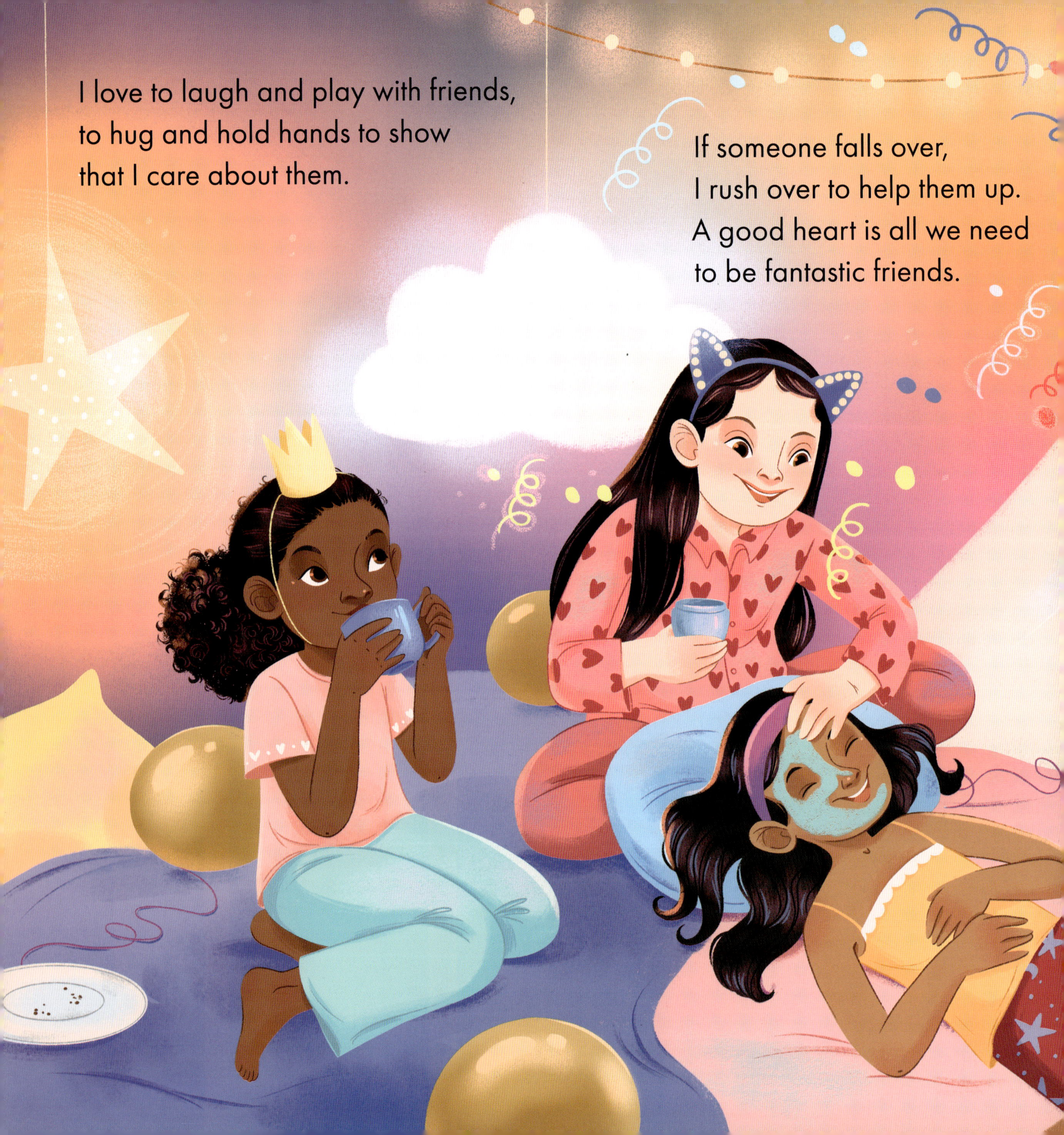

I love to laugh and play with friends,
to hug and hold hands to show
that I care about them.

If someone falls over,
I rush over to help them up.
A good heart is all we need
to be fantastic friends.

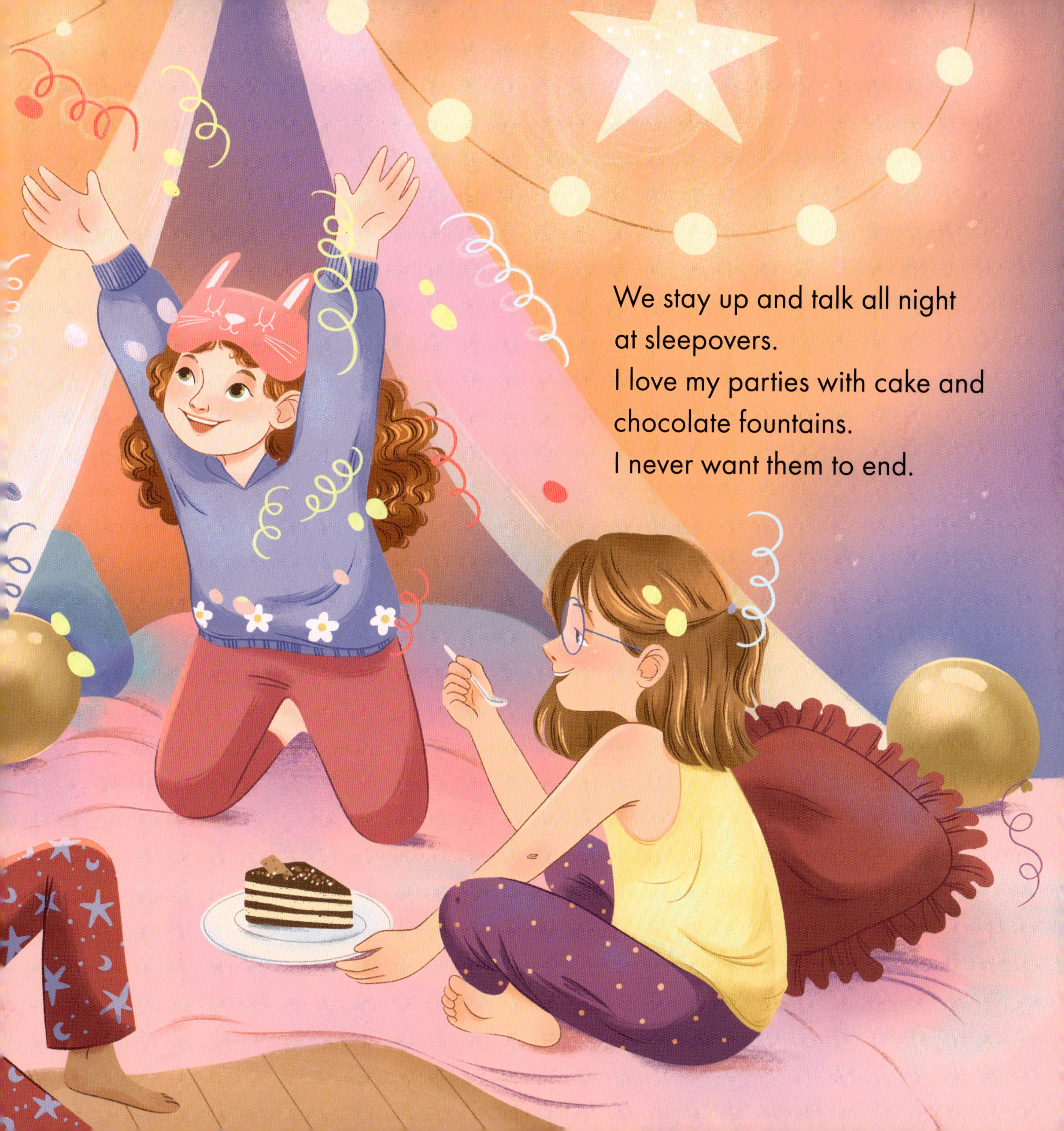

We stay up and talk all night
at sleepovers.
I love my parties with cake and
chocolate fountains.
I never want them to end.

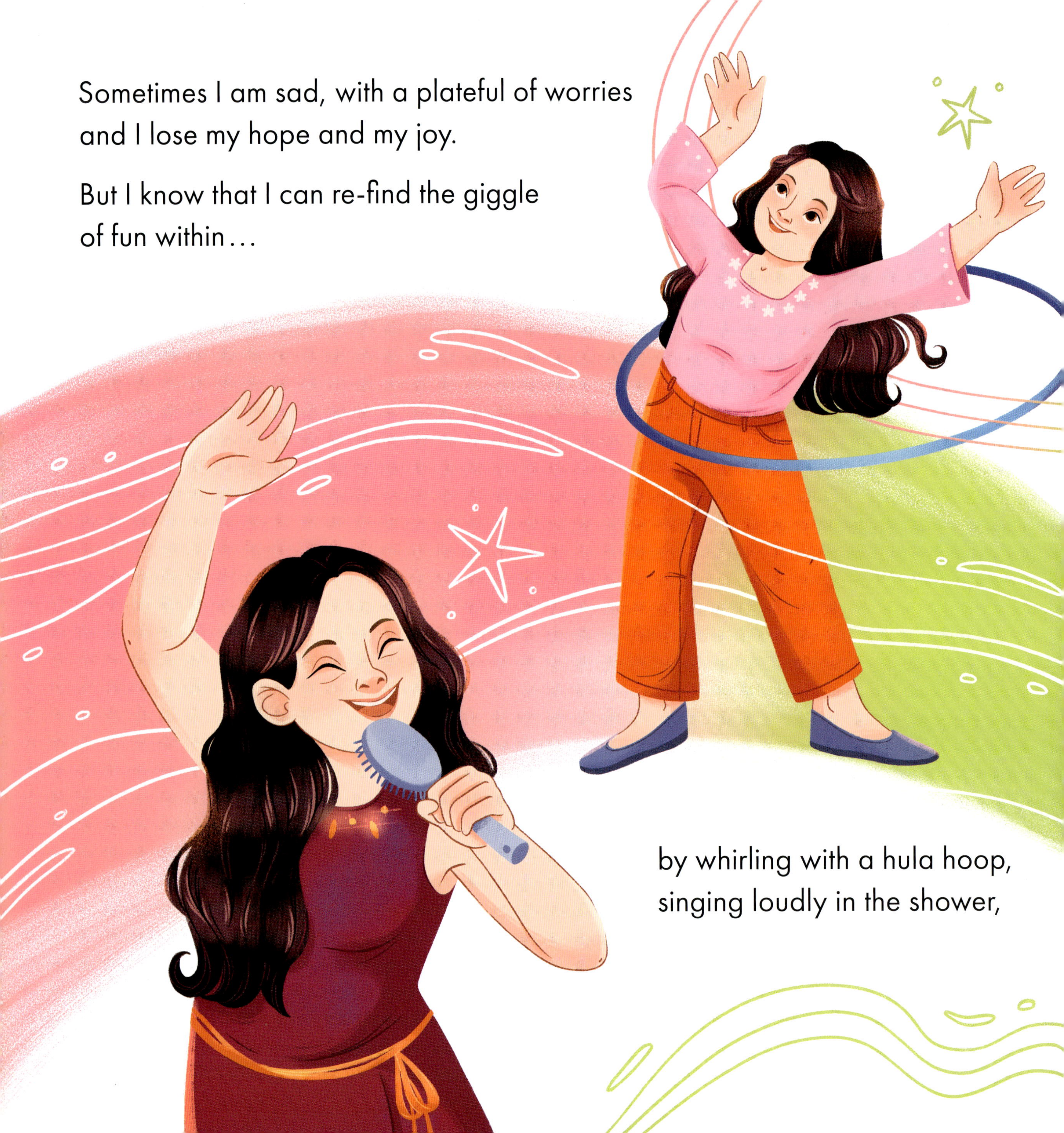

Sometimes I am sad, with a plateful of worries
and I lose my hope and my joy.

But I know that I can re-find the giggle
of fun within…

by whirling with a hula hoop,
singing loudly in the shower,

by taking deep breaths,
dancing to an upbeat song,

by talking and holding hands with a friend.

Why not try these things, too?

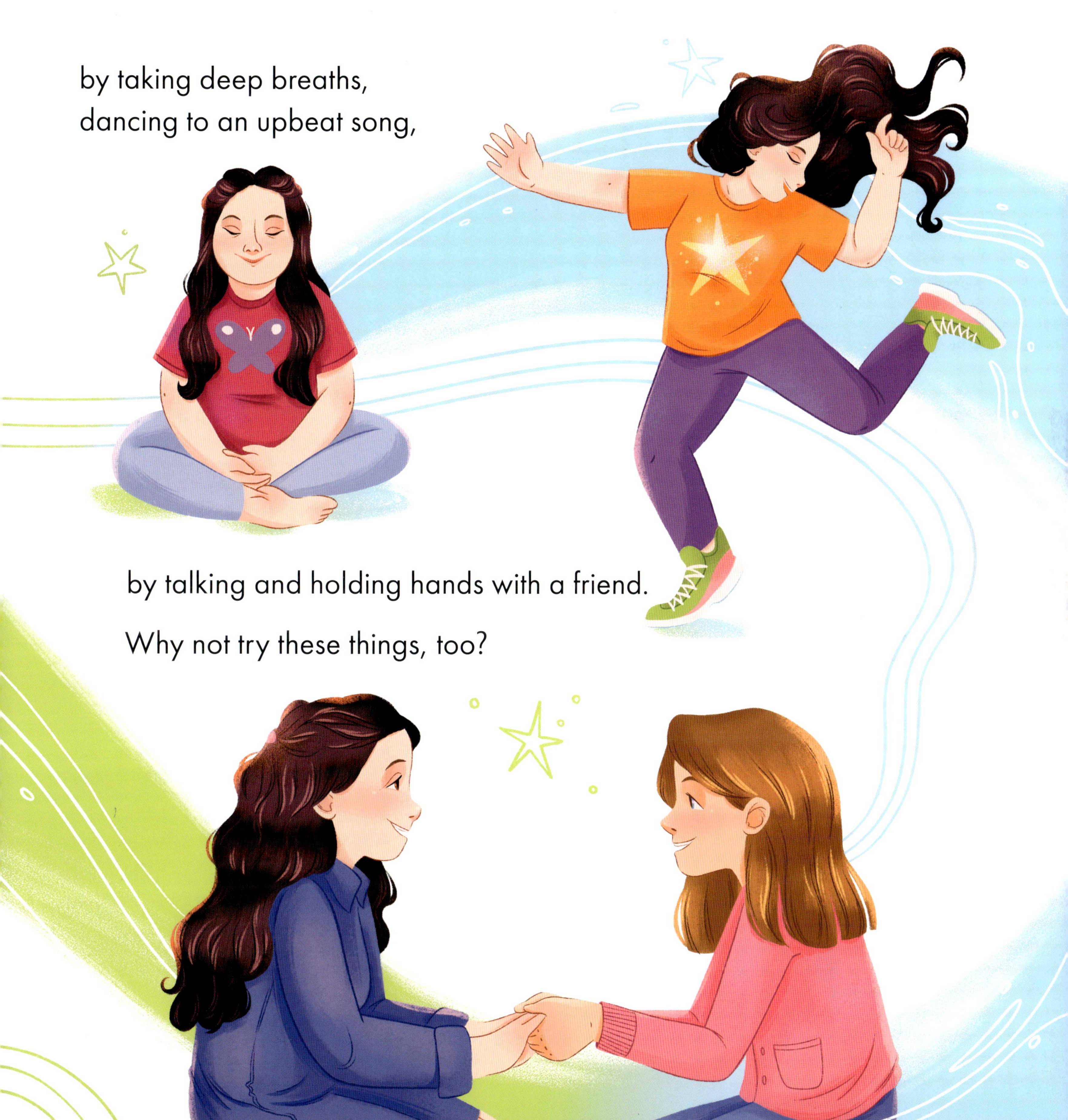

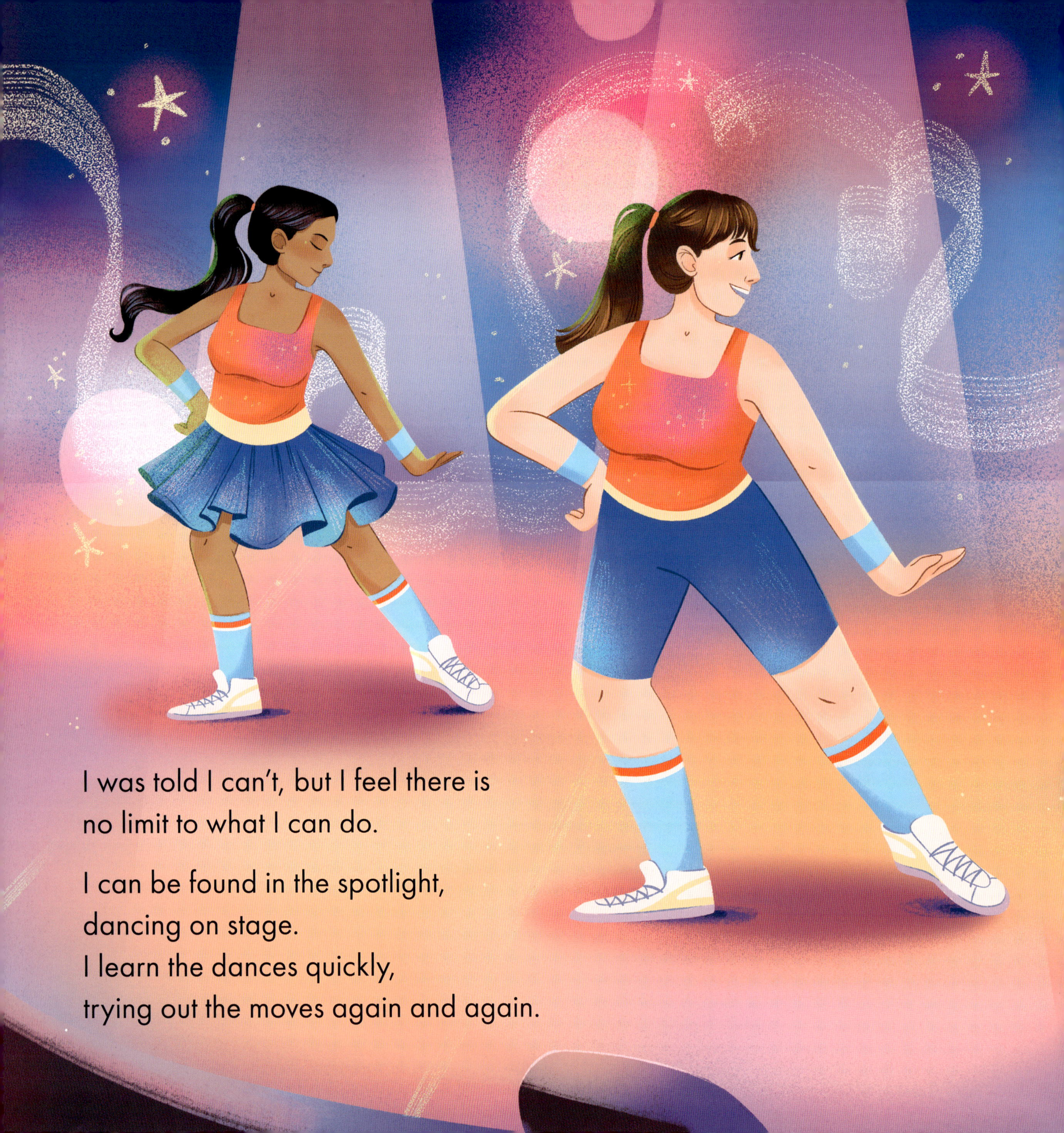

I was told I can’t, but I feel there is no limit to what I can do.

I can be found in the spotlight,
dancing on stage.
I learn the dances quickly,
trying out the moves again and again.

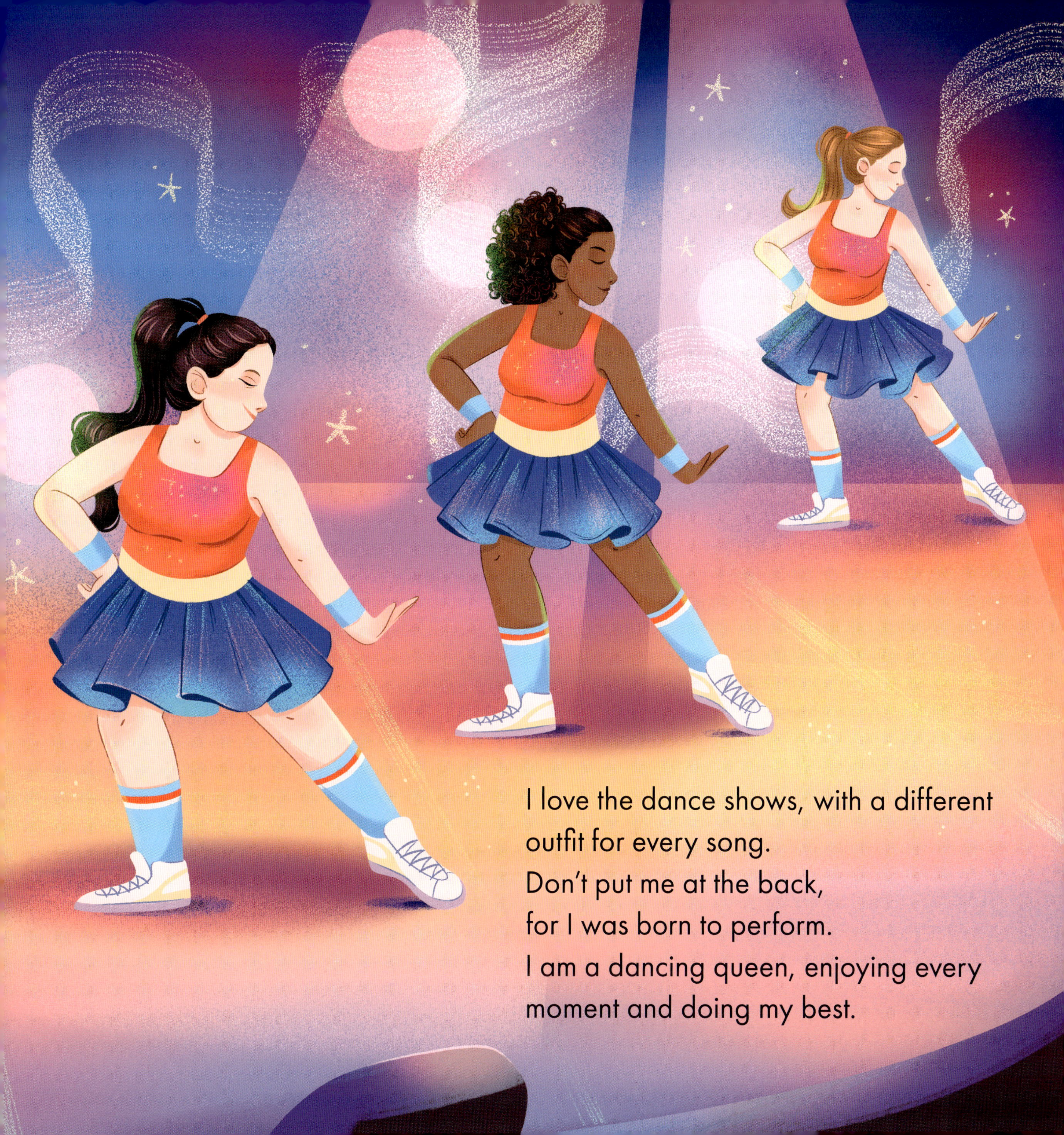

I love the dance shows, with a different
outfit for every song.
Don't put me at the back,
for I was born to perform.
I am a dancing queen, enjoying every
moment and doing my best.

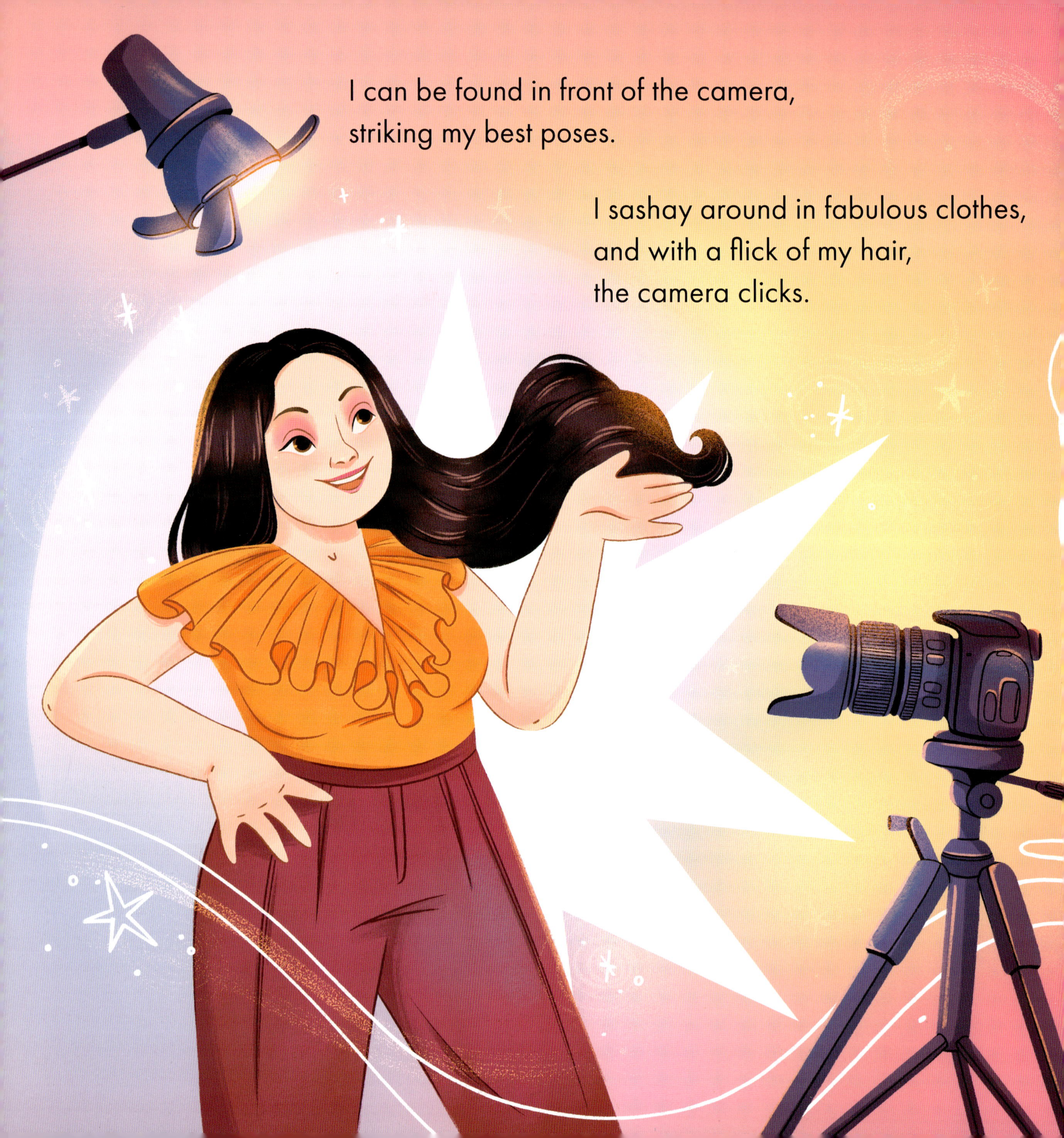

I can be found in front of the camera,
striking my best poses.

I sashay around in fabulous clothes,
and with a flick of my hair,
the camera clicks.

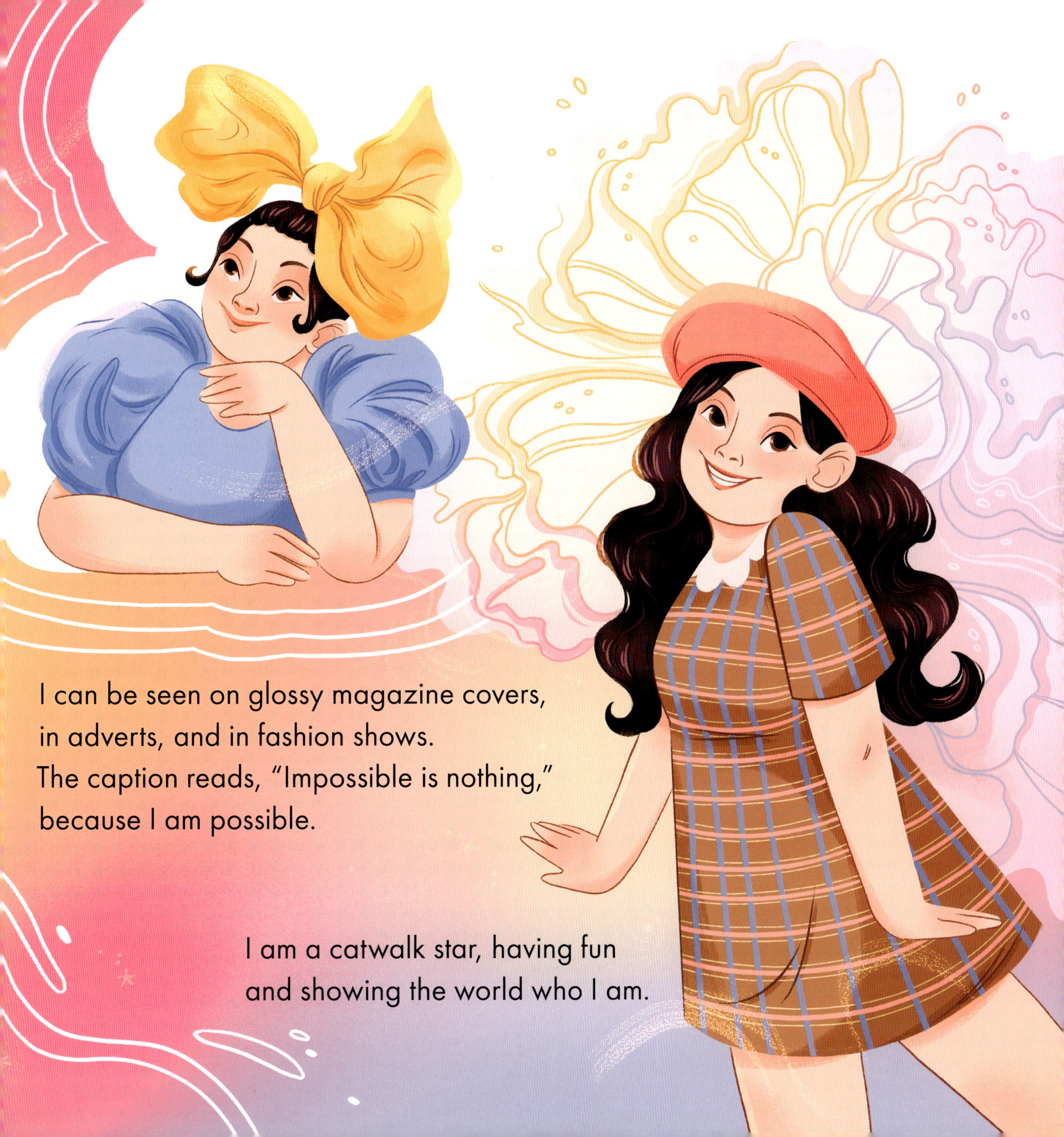

I can be seen on glossy magazine covers, in adverts, and in fashion shows. The caption reads, "Impossible is nothing," because I am possible.

I am a catwalk star, having fun and showing the world who I am.

I can be found on a painting in an art gallery and as a statue for all to see. There is even a doll that looks like people like me.

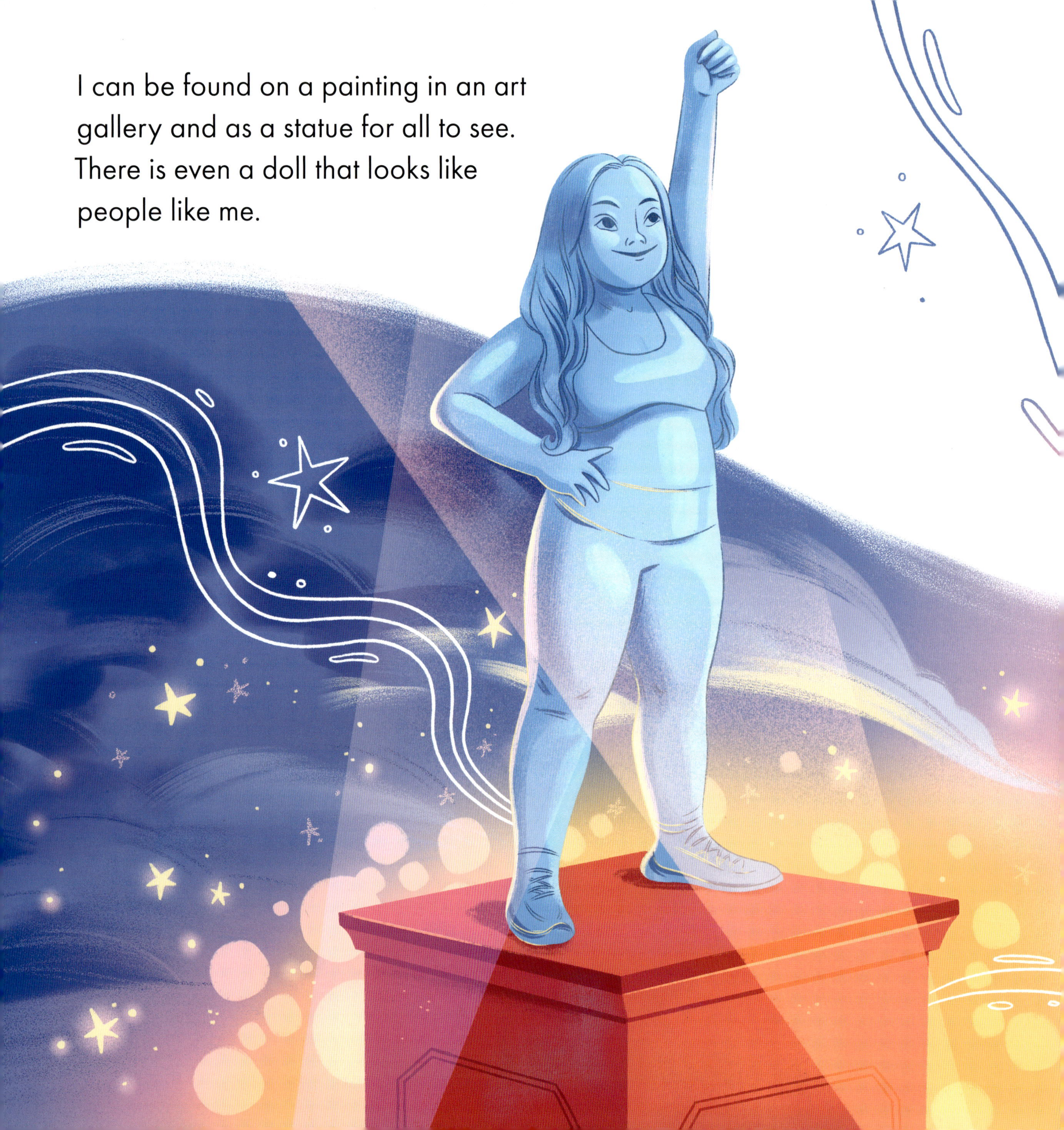

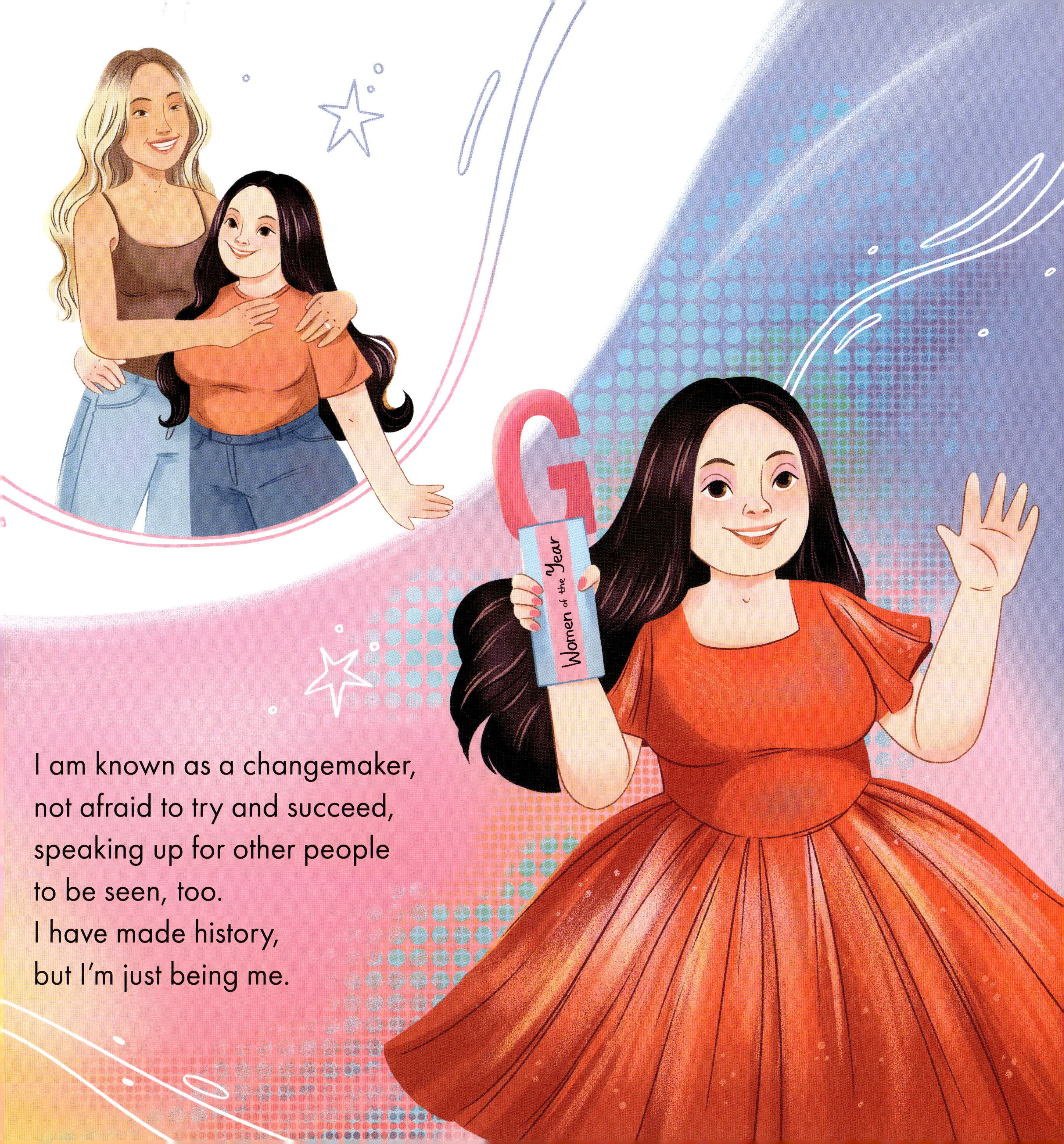

I am known as a changemaker,
not afraid to try and succeed,
speaking up for other people
to be seen, too.
I have made history,
but I'm just being me.

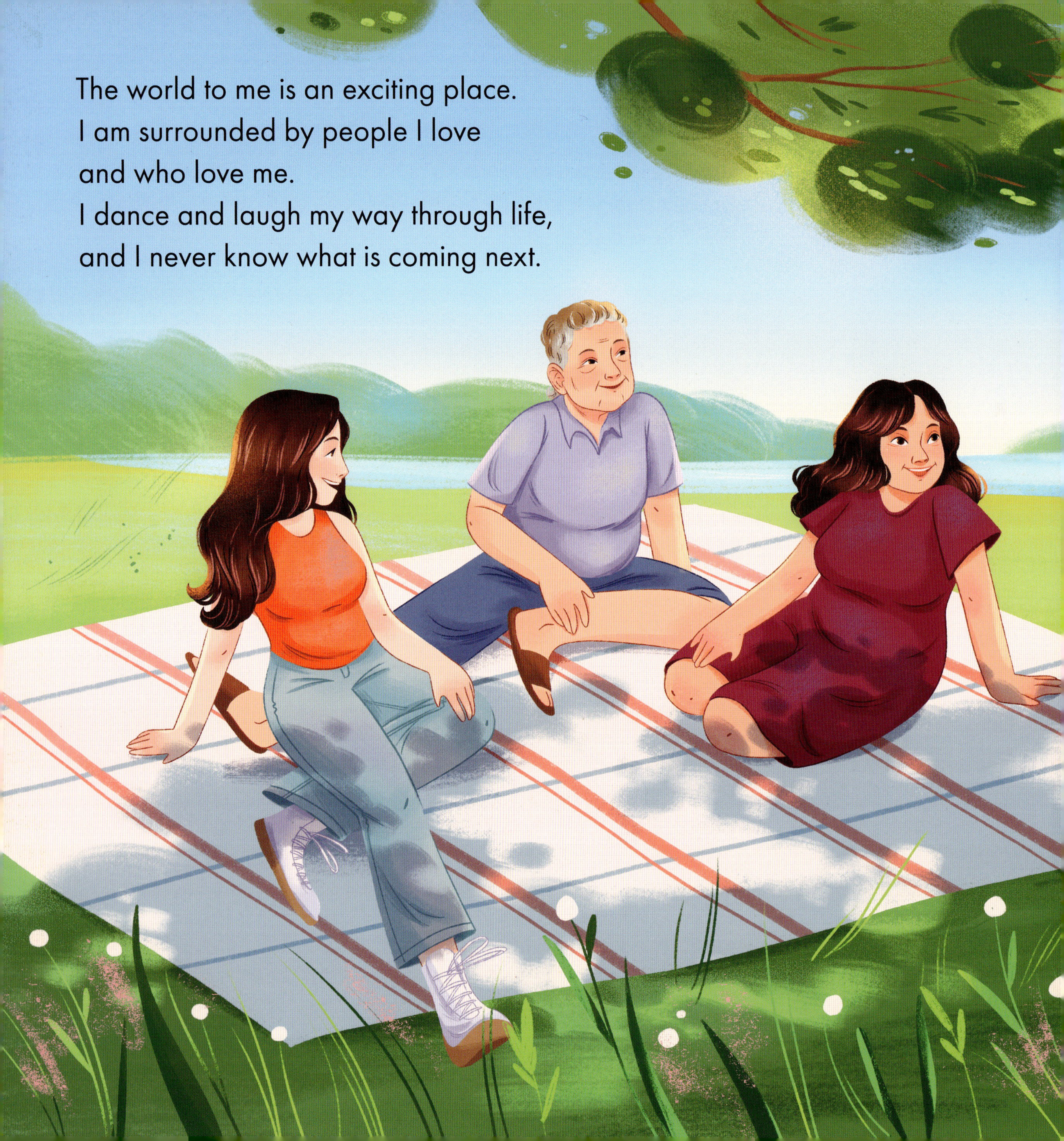

The world to me is an exciting place.
I am surrounded by people I love
and who love me.
I dance and laugh my way through life,
and I never know what is coming next.

You, too, can be excited by who you are and what you can do.
Try your best, and shine hope and joy all around.

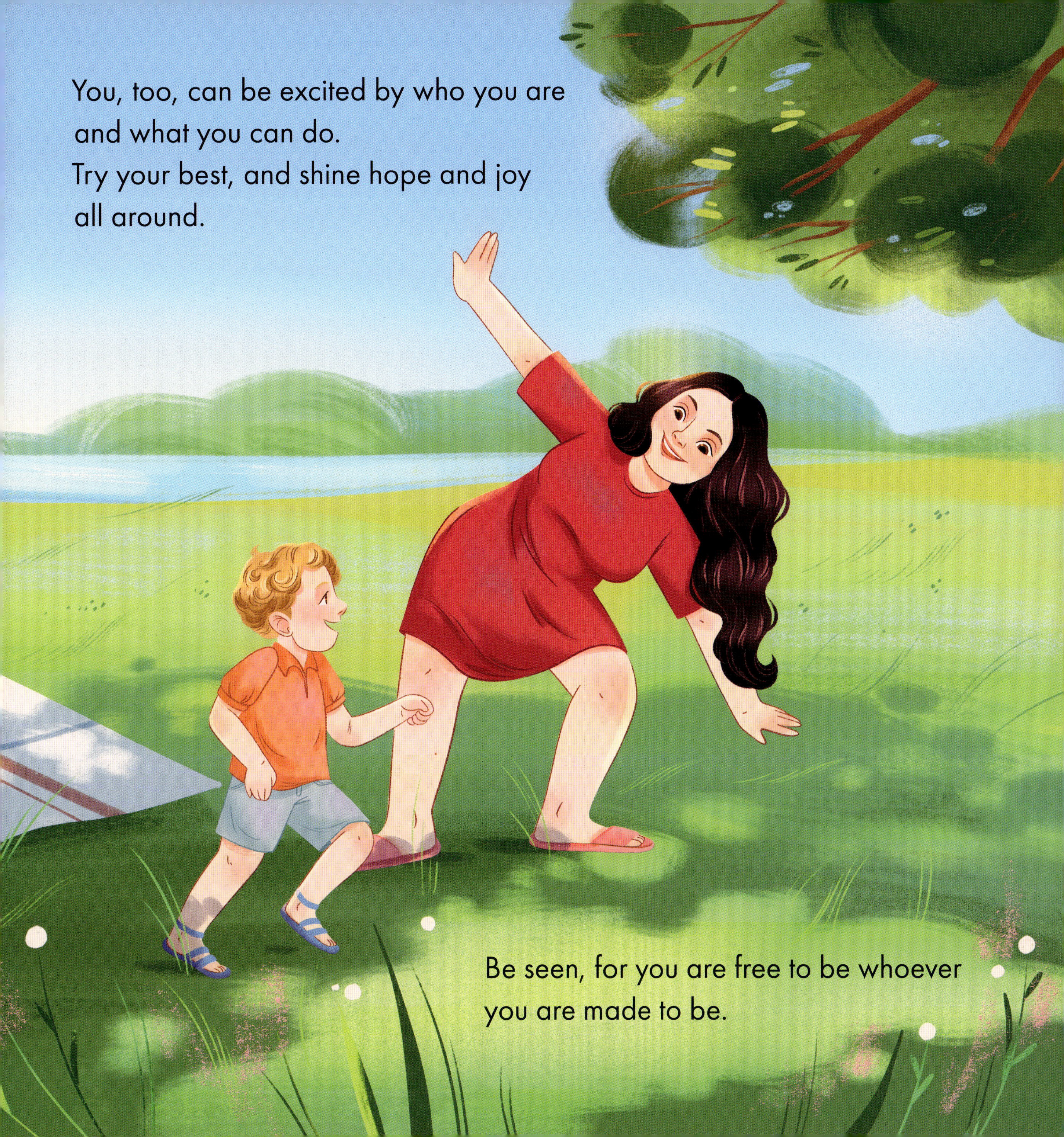

Be seen, for you are free to be whoever you are made to be.

Notes for parents and carers

Ellie was born with Down syndrome. This wasn't picked up during the pregnancy, so it was a bit of a shock. Down syndrome is a condition where the baby is born with one extra chromosome. One in every thousand babies in the UK is born with Down syndrome.

Our approach to bringing up Ellie was, **"Let's put Ellie first and her condition second!"** We just wanted to bring her up in the same way as we did our other daughter, Amy, who is eight years older than Ellie. We just took one day at a time, dealing with the stress, reviews, and meetings as they came up.

As with all people, everyone who has Down syndrome is different and has their own personality. They all learn at different levels and at different speeds, and are sometimes just a little slower in learning. Ellie showed her frustration when she couldn't immediately do everything she wanted to do, but we celebrated the manageable little steps. Ellie attended mainstream school up to the age of 13 with classroom-assistant support. She then attended a special needs school to gain her qualifications, and is now in her final year at mainstream college. With amazing support and Ellie's own determination to do her best, **Ellie has achieved so much in her life so far, and is living proof that having Down syndrome should never hold you back.**